I0469334

The
Compendium
of Infection Control Technologies

First Workbook Edition, Introduction

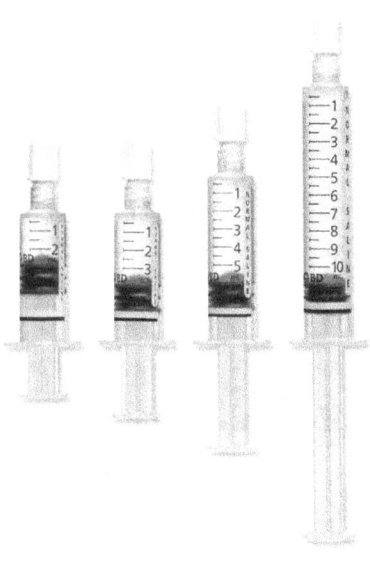

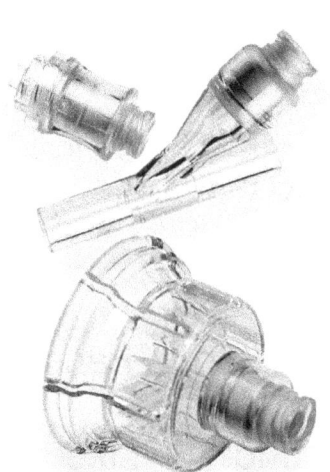

Consider the devices in this book and then order the literature and samples you need at:

www.MedicalSafetyBook.com

Get this introductory book for free.

I did not really want to charge for this introductory book.   Because of the printing and distribution costs with Amazon.com, I have to.

Feel free to use the following link to download free PDF versions of this intro and to distribute them freely to your colleagues and other departments.

First: Go to Facebook.com/MedicalSafetyBook

Second: Like us on Facebook.

Then you will be directed to the download link for this introduction.

A link to download copies of this introductory PDF will appear in the links on that page.

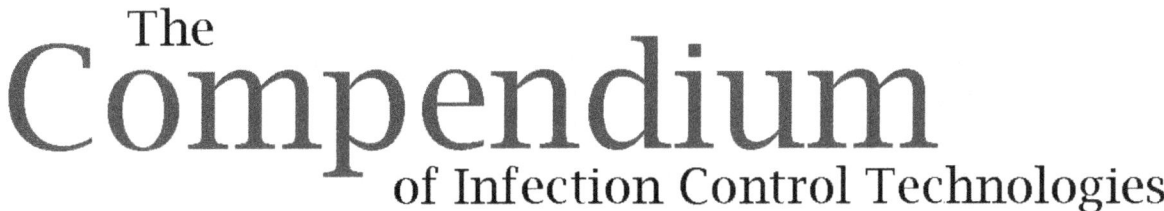

The Compendium
of Infection Control Technologies

INTRODUCTION

This workbook is designed to cut hundreds of man-hours off of the biomedical safety device evaluation portion of the task of creating an Exposure Control Plan.

In 2010, the incidence of needlestick injuries in the United States, alone, was about 384,000, as estimated by the CDC. Most needlestick injuries result from hollow bore disposable syringes and needles. Even though most needlestick injuries do not result in serious infection, they often inflict severe psychological damage on the injured employee. Waiting months or more after an injury, just waiting and waiting for one to find out if they have contracted HIV or one of the Hepatitis Viruses, can be devastating.

By using the proper safety devices, most of these injuries could have been prevented. The safe handling and disposal of needles and other sharp instruments must be a priority for all health care providers. This is not only to protect health care workers but to protect employers as well.

In the US, OSHA mandates that every employer, where even a single employee is at risk of possible exposure to infection via contaminated sharps, must have a written exposure control plan in place. As part of this plan, every engineering control and medical device designed to prevent such an incident must be evaluated for appropriateness for sharps injury prevention. The results of each evaluation must be maintained in written form and kept on the premises and made available to OSHA in the event of an inspection.

Why you should have your plan in place:

An Exposure Control Plan must be in place in every facility. Besides the obvious benefit of dramatically increasing employee safety, failure to have such a plan in place creates several major liabilities for health care facilities, all employers with at-risk employees, and of course, the employees. These liabilities include, but are certainly not limited to:

- ....Possible of sharps injuries
- ....OSHA actions in the event of an inspection. OSHA fines for failure to comply often rise to the level of six figures, sometimes 7 (really).

☐ .... Employee legal actions that may follow an employee's sharps injury that could have been prevented, especially when there is an incomplete or no plan in place the might have prevented that accident.

Audit data suggests that of the occupational injuries that occur in hospitals, 16% are attributable to sharps injuries. (National Audit Office. The management of medical equipment in acute NHS Trusts in England, HCP 475 Session 1998–1999. London: Stationery Office; 1999. (Guideline Ref ID NAO1999).

As of 2003, it was estimated that needlestick injuries in the United States resulted in over 1000 Hepatitis B, Hepatitis C, and HIV infections in healthcare workers. Most, if not all, of these injuries could have been prevented.

All sharps injuries are considered to be potentially preventable. The preventability of such events are what puts the employer at risks. An employer who had ignored mandated procedures for sharps injury prevention would be in a poor position to defend itself from a lawsuit filed by an employee who had contracted a serious, or potentially lethal, injury, especially when they were using a non-safety device, rather than a properly evaluated safety device that could have potentially prevented the injury.

Can you afford a $100,000 fine?

OSHA requires that each facility seek out and evaluate all the medical devices on the market which are designed for the prevention of sharps injuries. The task is enormous and the fines for non-compliance often exceed $100,000. How often is often? In 2010, often was 164 times. Fines exceeding $100,000 were levied more than three times every week of the year.

Most of the devices that are listed in this compendium are currently available worldwide. Some may have already been discontinued or superseded. Let us know if you find either of these states to be true. More devices are available and our research is ongoing to provide you with access to additional devices as they become available. Updates to this publication will be made available at least once a year.

Best use of this publication:

After looking through each volume of this Compendium Workbook, you will need to choose which devices to evaluate. Go to MedicalSafetyBook.Com/signup.php and join for free.

Then click on the BROWSE SAMPLES link & order (usually free) samples of all of the devices you wish to pursue. Don't be shy; The manufacturers want to hear from you and give you the opportunity to choose their devices.

When you get your samples:

In your workbook, each safety device is paired with an evaluation form that will facilitate rapid evaluation of that device.   Look at the forms for each of the devices that you wish to evaluate. Make changes to the form if you feel you need to to make it conform to the specific needs of your facility. Use a different form if that works better for you. Email us if you need a digital copy of any of the forms so that you can revise it to conform to your facility's needs.

Printed version

This printed version is designed to be used as a safety device evaluation workbook. Once completed, the printed edition can be placed on your shelf to be presented to OSHA in the event of an inspection.

Please note, this notebook is only one part of your infection control plan and completing a thorough medical safety device evaluation and infection prevention plan, tailored to your facility's needs, remains your responsibility. No form will be perfect for every facility. Make changes to the forms and make them work for you.

This workbook is designed to replace many hundreds of man-hours of labor and many thousands of dollars of expenses that are involved in creating your exposure control plan.

If one nurse spent as little as two weeks working on this section of the ECP, it would cost, (with the average salary for registered nurses at about $40 per hour), it would cost about $3200. With this book, the savings would be more than $3000.00. And, by the way, it can't be done in two weeks. It can't be done in four weeks, either. Maybe 4 months. No, probably not.

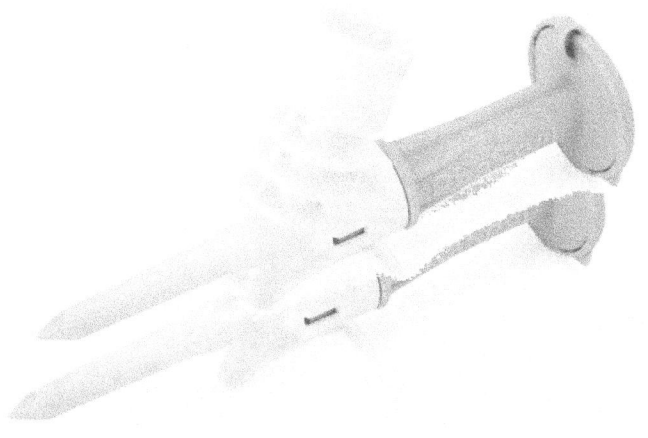

The Compendium
of Infection Control Technologies

First Workbook Edition, Book 2

Foreword

By Joel S. Rossen DVM

This book was created out of necessity. Initially, my necessity, now yours. As a small manufacturer of medical devices for nearly 20 years, my experience had been restricted to development and manufacturing of electronic stimulation devices for the treatment of pain and retinal dysfunctions, such as macular degeneration. My first patent, for the MicroStim, our flagship electical stimulator, was allowed in 1991.

A decade later, when my focus turned towards manufacturing of sharps safety devices, I created Biomedical Safety Technologies, LLC. The mission of BST was to provide bandages with unique properties to assist healthcare workers in bandaging injections sites with one hand, while minimizing exposure to bloodborne pathogens and maintaining possession of contaminated sharps. While these devices, known as Preemptive Dressings™ are not currently on the market, I decided to leave them in this publication in case some company out there decides they would like to license and market them. Seriously, although, I initially created this book so my company could afford to swim in a bigger pond. Now, it has taken on a life of its own.

By dressing an injection site prior to penetrating the skin, prolonged possession of a contaminated sharp becomes unnecessary. We coined and trademarked the term, Preemptive Dressings™ as a name for a type of dressing that was designed to preempt sharps injuries.

Please see more about the Preemptive Dressings is in Book 3, Chapter 7 of this workbook edition.

Even with such a great idea, we found that entering the marketplace was cost prohibitive. How could a company our size (tiny) spread the word in such a massive industry where a page or two of advertising costs exceeded our manufacturing and R & D budgets combined?

Meanwhile, OSHA revised the Bloodborne Pathogen Standard in response to the Needlestick Safety and Prevention Act of 2000. Enforcement of that standard has been steadily increasing since implementation of the new standard. Every facility with even one employee at risk for exposure to blood or other potentially infectious materials (OPIM) is subject to the new standard. A tremendous regulatory burden has been placed on facilities where exposure to blood or pathogens is a known risk. For small practices, compliance may be nearly impossible.

Interestingly, the fact that we, Biomedical Safety Technologies, LLC, have not been advertising our Preemptive Dressing does not excuse employers subject to "The Standard" from locating and evaluating our devices. Fair or not, until now, there has not been any comprehensive publication nor central source for listing and evaluating exposure control devices. While there are a multitude of engineering controls designed specifically to make healthcare workers safer, finding them has been hit and miss and is largely a matter of luck and very long hours, and that is before the procurement and evaluation processes even begin.

Because of the Bloodborne Pathogen Standard (BPS), healthcare facilities are now taxed to locate, evaluate, or at least consider, every medical device or engineering control that is available for infection control. And, as if evaluation of these devices was not difficult enough, locating and identifying the devices can be just as difficult. A small facility could expect to put an extra nurse on full-time just to locate the devices that they had to then evaluate.

On the other side of that void were companies like mine. Small manufacturers of medical devices have been unable to create enough of a presence in the medical literature to be found by the very medical facilities that are required by law to evaluate their devices. There was no central source where a healthcare facility could go to see what was on the market.

I finally surmised that the only way Biomedical Safety Technologies could ever be big enough to be noticed was to become the source of information about safer medical devices. That is how and why this book was born. To create the book, I first explained to my wife that she could expect to be a widow for the next year or two. However grudgingly, she gave me her blessing.

Next, I contacted my son, Brent Rossen, to organize a software company and create a website where medical device companies could upload their sharps safety products into the format that you will see in the medical device section of this book. Brent teamed with programmers Nicole Beguesse and Jared Freedland to create an interactive website that has functioned almost flawlessly since it first went live.

Then I contacted my friend, Ron Stoker, Executive Director of ISIPS, the International Sharps Injury Prevention Society, to be my liaison to the sharps safety industry and co-author. Bringing Ron and Brent's team onto the Compendium team may have been the best decisions I have ever made, for without them, this device evaluation system could have never happened.

Ron and I then began an e-mail and telephone campaign to rally as many medical device manufacturers as possible. We soon found that the industry was very enthusiastic about our project. The result, so far, is that over 110 medical device companies have joined us to help create this book for you. New companies and additional subsidiaries of member companies have been joining our effort at the rate of about 2 to 3 each week. That is important to you, because by the time this book is in your hand, it will already need updating. But, not to worry, that's a good thing. As a companion to this book, we have created, MedicalSafetyBook.com.

Your book comes with a free membership to MedicalSafetyBook.com. MedicalSafetyBook.com will be your continuing source for access to new safer medical devices as they become available.

Once you join MedicalSafetyBook.Com (for free), you will be notified by e-mail whenever a new device becomes available. You won't happen upon it in some obscure journal several days after an OSHA inspector comes knocking on your door .... you will know first. You will be able to keep your sharps safety plan up-to-date with the confidence that you are aware of and have considered at least most of the devices that can make your facility safer. For our part, we will continue our effort to place every known safer medical device in our book or on the website.

In addition to email notifications, printed supplements to this book will be published every time an additional (approximately) 100 devices are added to the database. In the printed editions and supplements, each device is paired with an evaluation form. You can perform your medical device evaluations in the notebook and then place it on the shelf as part of your formal Exposure Control Plan.

Why You Need This Device Evaluation System

By law, you are responsible to procure and test the devices. Out of the two hundred and fifty or more devices in the book, you may elect to procure and evaluate 50% or more of them.

Simply making the phone calls to procure just a few of these devices would take hours or days. But, by going to MedicalSafetyBook.com, finding the devices you are interested in and clicking " ADD TO CART" an email will be sent directly to a pre-arranged representative at each of the manufacturers to procure your samples for evaluation. Ordering samples through our sample procurement center will save you weeks of phone calls. It can be completed in minutes and it costs you nothing.

In 2000, President Clinton signed the Needlestick Safety and Prevention Act into law. The Act forever changed the way medical devices were to be chosen for inclusion in medical practices. No longer can price, purchasing groups, or preferred suppliers be the final determining factor in choosing sharps and sharps injury prevention products. The Bill dictated that the safety of the healthcare provider must come first. It is no longer up to the employer whether or not to provide safer medical devices. The ACT and OSHA have already made that decision; Safer medical devices will be made available. The choice is now which ones to choose. Safety trumps price.

I have seen financial formulas that dictate how to balance the cost of medical devices against the safety of the provider. While some sources claim that if the safer device costs too much more than its conventional counterpart, it does not have to be incorporated into the sharps safety program, this is not the case.

You will not be excused just because your purchasing organization does not provide certain devices. Also, OSHA does not accept the failure of a purchasing organization to make safer medical devices available as a valid reason not to have those devices available in facilities that are required to adhere to the standard. If your purchasing group does not make the devices available that you need to make your workplace safer, you still need to find them and bring them in for evaluation. By themselves, the costs of safer medical devices are also not a valid consideration for rejecting those devices. Devices must be selected based on employee feedback. They must be evaluated for appropriateness in each facility and for each procedure for effectiveness in preventing occupational exposures to blood and other potentially infectious materials.

Note the interaction between Audrey Taffet of Terumo Medical Corporation and Richard Fairfax of OSHA.

In July, 2002, Ms. Audrey Taffet of Terumo Medical Corporation, wrote to OSHA for clarification of the standard in respect to cost and purchasing agreements. Richard E. Fairfax, Director, Directorate of Enforcement Programs, responded with the letter that follows.

Ms. Audrey Taffet   November 21, 2002

Manager, Business Development
Terumo Medical Corporation
2101 Cottontail Lane
Somerset, NJ 08873

Dear Ms. Taffet:

Thank you for your July 2002 letter to the Occupational Safety and Health Administration (OSHA) regarding the application of the requirement in the Bloodborne Pathogens Standard (29 CFR 1910.1030) to use safer medical devices, specifically for facilities working under Group Purchasing Organization (GPO) contracts. This letter constitutes OSHA's interpretation only of the requirements discussed and may not be applicable to any question not delineated within your original correspondence. Your letter is paraphrased below followed by OSHA's response.

We (Terumo) understand that the evaluation of new sharps safety devices should be conducted by frontline healthcare workers. Many healthcare facilities operate under a Group Purchasing Organization (GPO) contact, intended to organize purchasing and availability of medical supplies. The GPOs typically offer little, if any, variation with regard to needlestick safety products. In light of the OSHA requirements to use safer medical devices dependent on an evaluation performed by healthcare workers, GPOs should not restrict the selection and evaluation of such products. What is OSHA's viewpoint on this?

Your interpretation is correct. Devices must be selected based on employee feedback (29 CFR 1910.1030(c)(1)(v)). They must be evaluated for appropriateness for each procedure and effectiveness in preventing occupational exposures to blood and other potentially infectious materials (OPIM). If the availability and variety of devices is restricted, the employer may be in violation of the requirements: (1) to review and update the exposure control plan to reflect changes in technology that eliminate or reduce exposure to blood and OPIM (29 CFR 1910.1030(c)(1)(iv)(A)); (2) to review and update the plan annually, documenting the consideration and implementation of appropriate commercially available and effective safer medical devices designed to eliminate or minimize occupational exposure (29 CFR 1910.1030(c)(i)(iv)(B); and (3) to use engineering controls to eliminate or minimize employee exposure (29 CFR 1910.1030(d)(2)(i)).

Remember, selecting a safer device based solely on the lowest cost is not appropriate. Selection must be based on employee feedback and device effectiveness. OSHA compliance officers have issued citations to employers at facilities that were not using effective engineering controls because of the product availability limits of their purchasing contracts. Again, if during an OSHA inspection, it is determined that an employer did not evaluate and select appropriate and effective devices, the employer may be cited. In an effort to best serve the safety and regulatory needs of their clients, GPOs should offer a variety of different safer devices.

Thank you for your interest in occupational safety and health. We hope you find this information helpful. OSHA requirements are set by statute, standards, and regulations. Our interpretation letters explain these requirements and how they apply to particular circumstances, but they cannot create additional employer obligations. This letter constitutes OSHA's interpretation of the requirements discussed. Note that our enforcement guidance may be affected by changes to OSHA rules. Also, from time to time we update our guidance in response to new information. To keep apprised of such developments, you can consult OSHA's website at http://www.osha.gov. If you have any further questions, please feel free to contact the Office of Health Enforcement at (202) 693-2190.

Sincerely,
Richard E. Fairfax, Director
Directorate of Enforcement Programs

Even if it weren't for the hundreds or thousands of injuries annually; Even if it weren't for the shattered families and psyches;this one small letter, by itself, would be more than sufficient justification for any practice to acquire this book and fully implement a comprehensive written exposure control plan. Sharps safety programs save lives.

When you perform your evaluations, we strongly suggest that each practice go beyond the simple completion of the evaluation forms and establish scenarios and criteria not only for the practice in general, but for the various different procedures within the practice. In a multi-disciplinary practice, you are likely to find that you need this book for a number of departments around the facility, and that a single ECP will not suffice for the whole facility.

Sharps safety requirements can differ profoundly from one procedure to the next; A device chosen as the safest alternative for one aspect of your practice may not fare so well in another department. Be sure you consider every possible variable in creating, documenting, and implementing your sharps safety program.

You can e-mail your suggestions to suggestions@medicalsafetybook.com. They may or may not be implemented, but they will always be read and seriously considered.

We present this book to you with respect and sincere thanks for allowing us to participate at a level where we can truly make a difference.

Thank you for welcoming our book into your practice. Our sincere wish is that you derive benefit many, many, times greater than your investment.

Sincerely

Joel Rossen DVM

Introduction to the

The Compendium of Infection Control Technologies' Safety Device Evaluation Workbook

(To Assist in the Development of Your Exposure Control Plan)

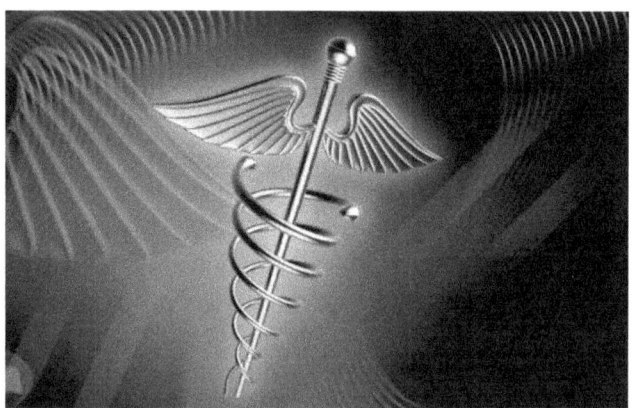

Just Answer One Simple Question to Decide If You Need This Workbook

Please answer this question:

Do you have at least **one** employee that is at risk of being exposed to bloodborne pathogens by a sharps injury?

YES or NO ?

If you answered YES, and you do not have an up-to-date, completed Exposure Prevention Plan (ECP), then you must purchase and use this workbook.

Avoid massive OSHA fines. Fines for failure to comply with the OSHA's BPS (Bloodborne Pathogen Standard) **often** exceed $100,000.00. How often is often? In 2010, fines exceeding six figures were levied by OSHA more than three times per week (164 times during that one year).

What is this book?

It is a workbook designed to facilitate and streamline the safety medical device evaluation section of your ECP. It presents nearly 300 medical devices (engineering controls) and pairs each with a form to perform a systematic written evaluation of those devices. This workbook, once completed, becomes an integral part of your ECP.

Who created this publication?

I am sure you are wondering where this set of workbooks was developed. It is a cooperative effort led by Dr. Joel Rossen, Director of MedicalSafetyBook.com and Ron Stoker, Executive Director of ISIPS -- The International Sharps Injury Prevention Society, with the assistance of these organizations:

NAPPSI - The National Alliance for the Primary Prevention of Sharps Injuries

Premier - The Premier Safety Institute

AOHP - Association of Occupational Health Professionals

MIC - Managing Infection Control Magazine

TDICT - Training for Development of Innovative Control Technology Project (evaluation forms)

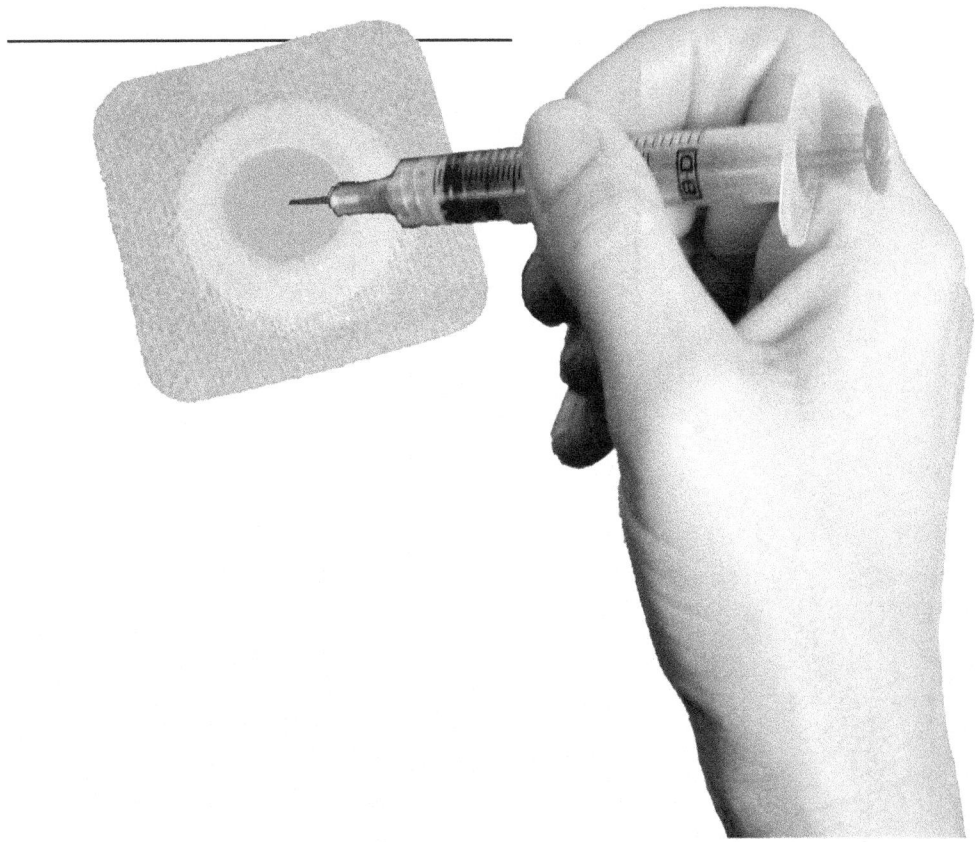

Contributors

We, Joel Rossen and Ron Stoker, wish to thank and acknowledge the organizations on the following pages for their unselfish assistance in the compilation of the Compendium.

Medical and Occupational Safety Organizations and Medical Infection Control Publications

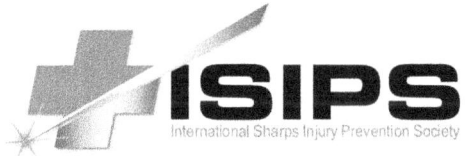

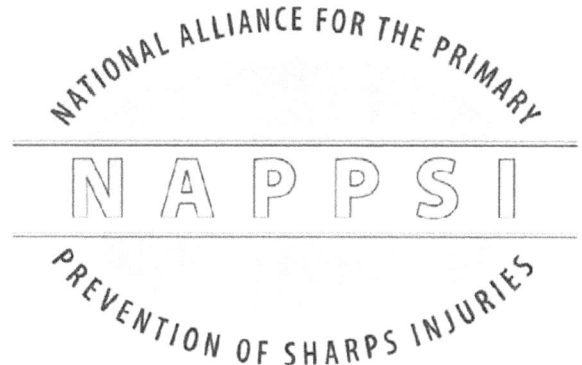

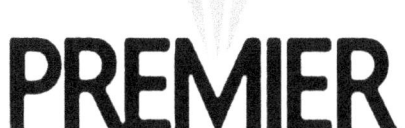

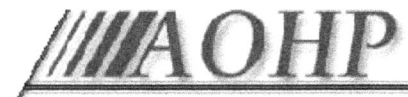

How Will this Workbook Help You Survive an OSHA Audit?

We can't promise that it actually will. But we can promise that having an extensive device evaluation and consideration section for your ECP, as required by the Bloodborne Pathogen Standard, will work to your advantage.

OSHA requires that every business facility, medical or otherwise, with even a single employee at risk of bloodborne pathogen exposure, must have a written exposure control plan (ECP) in place. That plan must include consideration of evaluation of every safety device commercially available for the prevention of sharps injuries. The safety device evaluation portion of the plan is a gargantuan task, requiring many hundreds of man hours of research before device evaluations can even begin. It is so burdensome that many facilities, those that are required to have extensive safety device evaluations included in their Exposure Control Plans, find they are unable to complete it. They fail to complete it either because they do not have the time, the task is too overwhelming, or because they do not have the funds to do so.

In order to reduce or eliminate the hazards of occupational exposure to bloodborne pathogens, an employer must implement an exposure control plan (ECP) for the worksite with details on employee protection measures. The plan must describe how an employer will use a combination of engineering and work practice controls, ensure the use of personal protective clothing and equipment, provide training , medical surveillance, hepatitis B vaccinations, and signs and labels, among other provisions.

Engineering controls are the primary means of eliminating or minimizing employee exposure and include the use of safer medical devices, such as needleless devices, shielded needle devices, and plastic capillary tubes.

In October, 2010, Briefings on Infection Control reported that in 2009 and 2010, all five of the top most expensive OSHA violations included noncompliant exposure control plans and post exposure procedures.

Any sharps injury might trigger an OSHA inspection/audit. When OSHA inspects a facility and finds it non-compliant with terms of the bloodborne pathogen exposure prevention standards, the fines can be hefty. What is the first thing they look at when they inspect? Your Exposure Control Plan, of course. Lack of engineering and work practice controls and failure to update the ECP at least annually constitute the top deficiencies cited by OSHA.

What fines? In 2009, there were 120 cases with fines in excess of $100,000.00. Yes, in excess of six figures. In 2010, that number jumped by 37%, to 164.

What does this workbook provide?

This workbook bootstraps development of your ECP by cutting hundreds of hours off the preparation and evaluation time for engineering controls (safety products). It lists, with full page descriptions, nearly 300 different safety devices and engineering controls as a starting point for the device evaluation section of your ECP. In addition to photographs, each device has a text description, a paragraph of advantages (according to the manufacturer), a presentation of its safety features and benefits, a description of the mechanics, and links to the manufacturer so you can follow up if you choose to.

Each device is paired with an evaluation form, chosen by the manufacturer, to facilitate your evaluation of that device for your facility.

The following pages will reveal the heart of this workbook to you. Below are a several randomly chosen of examples of the devices presented along with their paired evaluation forms. The Compendium Workbook is your introduction to hundreds of devices and a headstart towards their evaluations

Notice that each of the forms contains a number of links to access the manufacturers of the devices. For your sample procurement, we invite you to use, MedicalSafetyDevice.com, free of charge, of course.

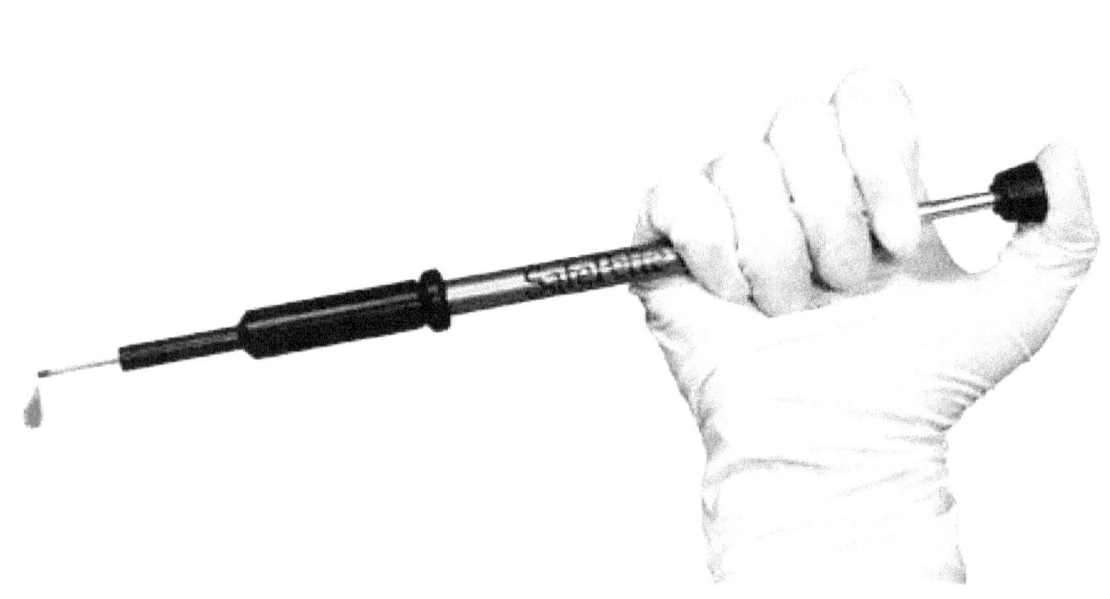

www.MedicalSafetyBook.com.

Haemo-Diff Blood Smear

Device Description:
Sarstedt's Haemo-Diff Blood Smear is designed specifically to work with the S-Monovette® Blood Collection System. The unique device creates a blood droplet directly from the closed S-Monovette® tube and smears this droplet onto the slide. This double function minimizes exposure to bloodborne pathogens and eliminates the need for additional products.

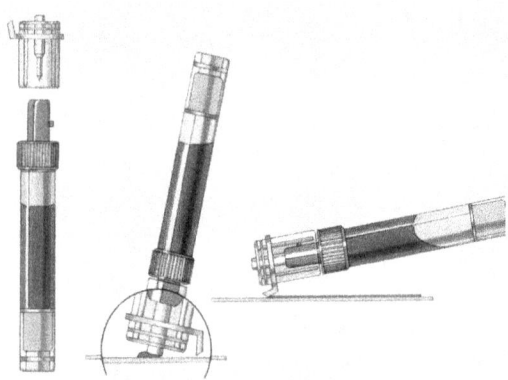

Advantages:
Place the Haemo-Diff vertically onto the S-Monovette®, piercing the membrane. Place the Haemo-Diff in a sloping position onto the slide to dispense a droplet of blood. Move the Haemo-Diff toward the droplet as usual to create a smear.

Safety Features and Benefits:
The Sarstedt Haemo-Diff minimizes exposure to bloodborne pathogens because opening of the tube is no longer required during slide preparation. The dual-function device also saves time and material costs.

FDA Status:	Listed
Sizes Available:	One size fits all S-Monovette® tubes
Product Website:	www.sarstedt.com/php/produktfamilie-darstellung.php?familie_id=112&seite=1
Brochure Download:	www.sarstedt.com/php/prospektanforderung.php?selected_gruppe_id=11
Instructional Website:	www.sarstedt.com/php/produktfamilie-darstellung.php?familie_id=112&seite=1
Instructional Video:	
Contact for Samples:	MedicalSafetyBook.com
Contact for Purchase:	(800) 257-5101; sarstedt@bellsouth.net; www.sarstedt.com/php/email.php
Availability:	Now available
Manufacturer:	Sarstedt, Inc. 1025 St. James Church Road P.O. Box 468 Newton, NC 28658 USA 800-257-5101 www.sarstedt.com sarstedt@bellsouth.net

SARSTEDT

Blood Collection Equipment

SAFETY FEATURE EVALUATION FORM
VACUUM TUBE BLOOD COLLECTION SYSTEMS

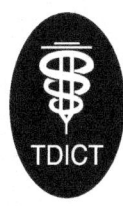

Date: _____ Department: _____ Occupation: _____

Product: _____ Number of times used: _____

Please **circle** the most appropriate answer for each question. Not applicable (N/A) may be used if the question does not apply to this particular product.

agree............disagree

1. The safety feature can be activated using a one-handed technique......................... 1 2 3 4 5 N/A
2. The safety feature **does not** interfere with normal use of this product..................... 1 2 3 4 5 N/A
3. Use of this product requires you to use the safety feature...................................... 1 2 3 4 5 N/A
4. This product **does not** require more time to use than a non-safety device.............. 1 2 3 4 5 N/A
5. The safety feature works well with a wide variety of hand sizes............................ 1 2 3 4 5 N/A
6. The safety feature works with a butterfly.. 1 2 3 4 5 N/A
7. A clear and unmistakable change (either audible or visible) occurs when the
    safety feature is activated.. 1 2 3 4 5 N/A
8. The safety feature operates reliably.. 1 2 3 4 5 N/A
9. The exposed sharp is blunted or covered after use and prior to disposal................ 1 2 3 4 5 N/A
10. The inner vacuum tube needle (rubber sleeved needle) **does not** present a
    danger of exposure... 1 2 3 4 5 N/A
11. The **product does** not need extensive training to be operated correctly................. 1 2 3 4 5 N/A

Of the above questions, which three are the most important to **your** safety when using this product?

Are there other questions which you feel should be asked regarding the safety/ utility of this product?

Hypodermic Needle-Pro® Device with Syringe

Device Description:
Hypodermic Needle-Pro® devices are available for a wide range of clinical applications involving hypodermic needles including: medication delivery via syringe injections or prefilled medication cartridges, TB testing, immunizations, insulin injections, allergy testing, as well as delivery of pain medication and local anesthetics. Hypodermic Needle-Pro® devices are available pre-attached to 1, 3, 5, 10 mL syringes for the ultimate in safety syringe convenience.

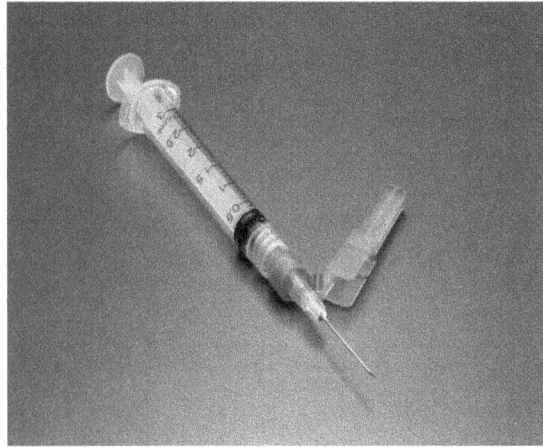

Advantages:
Hypodermic Needle-Pro® devices are available in needle gauge sizes 18 – 30g and in lengths ½" – 1 ½". 18 – 25g devices are ideal for intramuscular and subcutaneous injections, while 25 – 30g devices facilitate intradermal injections and do not contribute additional dead space to standard needle/syringe injections.

Safety Features and Benefits:
The Hypodermic Needle-Pro® device meets NIOSH/CDC recommendations for safety devices. Activation of the safety feature is similar to all Needle-Pro® devices, reducing training.

Mechanics:
The Hypodermic Needle-Pro® device is activated with a simple one-handed technique against any hard surface.

FDA Status:	Approved
Sizes Available:	1,3,5,10 mL; 20-27g Product
Website:	www.smiths-medical.com
Brochure Download:	www.smiths-medical.com
Instructional Website:	www.smiths-medical.com
Instructional Video:	www.smiths-medical.com
Contact for Samples:	www.MedicalSafetyBook.com
Contact for Purchase:	Phone:(800) 258-5361 Fax: (603) 352-3703
Availability:	Now available
Manufacturer:	Smiths Medical 10 Bowman Drive Keene, NH 03431 USA 800-258-5361 www.smiths-medical.com info@smiths-medical.com

Safety Syringe

smiths

SAFETY FEATURE EVALUATION FORM
SAFETY SYRINGES (and safety needles)

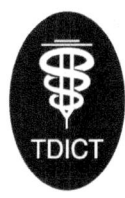

Date: —————— Department: —————————— Occupation: ——————————

Product: ——————————————————— Number of times used: ——————————

Please **circle** the most appropriate answer for each question. Not applicable (N/A) may be used if the question does not apply to this particular product.

DURING USE: agree............disagree

1. The safety feature can be activated using a one-handed technique............................1 2 3 4 5 N/A
2. The safety feature **does not** obstruct vision of the tip of the sharp.............................1 2 3 4 5 N/A
3. Use of this product requires you to use the safety feature...1 2 3 4 5 N/A
4. This product does not require more time to use than a non-safety device.................. 1 2 3 4 5 N/A
5. The safety feature works well with a wide variety of hand sizes................................ 1 2 3 4 5 N/A
6. The device is easy to handle while wearing gloves... 1 2 3 4 5 N/A
7. This device **does not** interfere with uses that do not require a needle.......................1 2 3 4 5 N/A
8. This device offers a good view of any aspirated fluid..1 2 3 4 5 N/A
9. This device will work with all required syringe and needle sizes............................... 1 2 3 4 5 N/A
10. This device provides a better alternative to traditional recapping.............................. 1 2 3 4 5 N/A

AFTER USE:

11. There is a clear and unmistakeable change (audible or visible) that occurs
    when the safety feature is activated.. 1 2 3 4 5 N/A
12. The safety feature operates reliably.. 1 2 3 4 5 N/A
13. The exposed sharp is permanently blunted or covered after use and prior to disposal.. 1 2 3 4 5 N/A
14. This device is no more difficult to process after use than non-safety devices........... 1 2 3 4 5 N/A

TRAINING:

15. The user **does not** need extensive training for correct operation............................. 1 2 3 4 5 N/A
16. The design of the device suggests proper use... 1 2 3 4 5 N/A
17. It is **not** easy to skip a crucial step in proper use of the device................................ 1 2 3 4 5 N/A

Of the above questions, which three are the most important to **your** safety when using this product?

Are there other questions which you feel should be asked regarding the safety/ utility of this product?

QlickSmart®

Device Description:
Single-handed scalpel blade removal, containment, and disposal system

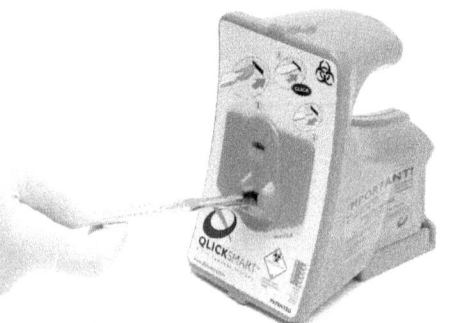

QlickSmart Blade Removal System

Advantages:
Allows Healthcare worker to continue using standard scalpel blade system and remain OSHA Compliant. Right or left handed use. Allows hands to remain behind sharp.

Safety Features and Benefits:
Makes removal of blade from handle very safe and reliable. Eliminates injuries to downstream staff.

Mechanics:
Handle with blade is inserted into front slot until a pronounced click is heard. Handle is then withdrawn from slot. The Qlicksmart has a built-in counter than counts down from 100 to 0, thereby indicating that Flask is full. The Qlicksmart Flask is then removed from reusable bracket and may be discarded in accordance to CDC Guidelines.

FDA Status:	Approved
Sizes Available:	Flask and Reusable Bracket
Product Website:	www.mycomedical.com
Brochure Download:	www.mycomedical.com
Instructional Website:	www.mycomedical.com
Instructional Video:	www.mycomedical.com
Contact for Samples:	Visit the Medical Safety Book.com Sample Procurement Center
Contact for Purchase:	Contact Customer Service at (800) 454-6926 to locate distributor.
Availability:	Now available
Manufacturer:	MYCO Medical 113 Centre West Court Cary, NC 27513 USA www.mycomedical.com sales@mycomedical.com

Scalpel Blade Remover

MYCO Medical
TheSharpChoice™

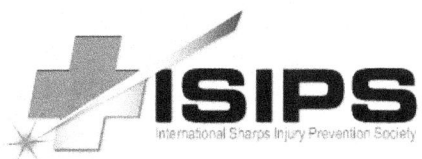

GENERIC SAFETY DEVICE EVALUATION FORM

Date: _____ Department: _____

Occupation: _____ Product: _____ Number of times used: _____

Please **circle** the most appropriate answer for each question. Not applicable (N/A) may be used if the question does not apply to this particular product.

		Agree.........Disagree
1	The use of the device does not require extensive change in technique.	1 2 3 4 5 N/A
2	This device provides a better alternative to non-safety product.	1 2 3 4 5 N/A
3	This device is no more difficult to use than traditional non-safety product and requires no additional time.	1 2 3 4 5 N/A
4	The device works well with a wide variety of hand sizes.	1 2 3 4 5 N/A
5	The device is easy to handle while wearing gloves.	1 2 3 4 5 N/A
6	The device can be used by either right or left handed clinicians.	1 2 3 4 5 N/A
7	The safety feature of the device does not cause interference with the procedure.	1 2 3 4 5 N/A
8	The user does not need extensive training for correct use of the product.	1 2 3 4 5 N/A
9	The product is suitable for a range of uses across a variety of patient populations.	1 2 3 4 5 N/A
10	The safety feature of the product is a passive feature; it requires no intervention on the part of the clinician to activate.	1 2 3 4 5 N/A
11	The user's hands are protected from a sharp at all times.	1 2 3 4 5 N/A
12	The device gives indication of safety feature activation.	1 2 3 4 5 N/A
13	The device provides audible and visual feedback that the safety feature has been activated.	1 2 3 4 5 N/A
14	The device has an undefeatable safety feature that provides permanent coverage of the sharp.	1 2 3 4 5 N/A
15	The device operates reliably.	1 2 3 4 5 N/A
16	The design of the product suggests proper use.	1 2 3 4 5 N/A
17	Use of the product requires you to use the safety feature.	1 2 3 4 5 N/A
18	Use of the product removes a sharp thus removing potential for exposure to sharps injury and bloodborne pathogen exposure.	1 2 3 4 5 N/A

Of the above questions, which three are the most important to your safety when using this product?

Are there other questions which you feel should be asked regarding the safety features of this product?

IonFusion Surgical Blade

Device Description:
The IonFusion Blade is the most rigorously tested blade on the market. The patented, golden edge IonFusion scalpel blades are manufactured from a high quality stainless steel. The IonFusion Blades have been bombarded with Zirconium Ions creating an edge that is twice as sharp as conventional blades carbon steel and stainlesss steel blades, and then placed in a heated annealing process that creates an edge that lasts 5 to 20 times as long as other conventional blades.

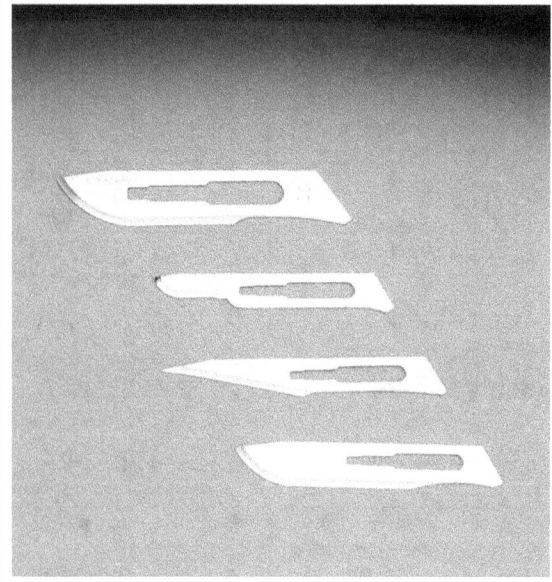

Advantages:
The IonFusion Surgical blade has been tested to be twice as sharp and 5 to 20 times longer lasting than compeititive conventional scalpel blades. The edge is gold to indicate quality and to signify that the physician is using an IonFusion Blade. The physician will be able to make finer incisions due to sharpness. The durability of the blade will cut down on blade usage and blade costs, and blade exchanges and changes between scrub nurse and physician.

Safety Features and Benefits:
The physician will be able to make finer incisions due to sharpness. The durability of the blade will cut down on blade usage, blade exchanges and changes between scrub nurse and physician, and blade count.

FDA Status:	Approved
Sizes Available:	#10, #11, #15, and #20 stainle
Product Website:	www.deroyal.com
Brochure Download:	www.deroyal.com
Instructional Website:	www.deroyal.com
Instructional Video:	www.deroyal.com
Contact for Samples:	Visit the Medical Safety Book.com Sample Procurement Center
Contact for Purchase:	Contact your local DeRoyal Area Manager or call DeRoyal Customer Service at 1-800-251-9864.
Availability:	Now available
Manufacturer:	DeRoyal Industries 200 DeBusk Lane Powell, TN 37849 USA 1-800-251-9864 www.deroyal.com jwalker@deroyal.com

Scalpel Blades

DeRoyal®

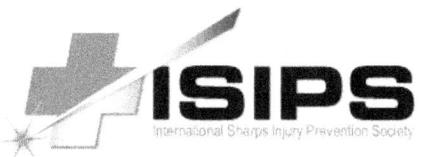

SAFETY SCALPEL EVALUATION FORM

Date: _____ Department: _____
Occupation: _____ Product: _____ Number of times used: _____

Please **circle** the most appropriate answer for each question. Not applicable (N/A) may be used if the question does not apply to this particular product.

		Agree.........Disagree
1	The safety feature of the scalpel can be activated using a one-handed technique.	1 2 3 4 5 N/A
2	The safety feature does not obstruct vision of the tip of the scalpel blade.	1 2 3 4 5 N/A
3	Use of this product requires you to use the safety feature.	1 2 3 4 5 N/A
4	This product does not require more time to use than a non-safety device.	1 2 3 4 5 N/A
5	The safety feature works well with a wide variety of hand sizes.	1 2 3 4 5 N/A
6	The device is easy to handle while wearing gloves.	1 2 3 4 5 N/A
7	This device provides a better alternative to traditional scalpels.	1 2 3 4 5 N/A
8	There is a clear and unmistakable change (audible or visible) that occurs when the safety feature is activated.	1 2 3 4 5 N/A
9	The safety feature operates reliably.	1 2 3 4 5 N/A
10	The safety feature has three positions: blade exposed, blade covered, blade permanently locked.	1 2 3 4 5 N/A
11	After being placed in the permanently locked position the safety feature cannot be undone.	1 2 3 4 5 N/A
12	This safety scalpel is no more difficult to use than non-safety scalpels.	1 2 3 4 5 N/A
13	The user does not need extensive training for correct use of the product.	1 2 3 4 5 N/A
14	The design of the product suggests proper use.	1 2 3 4 5 N/A
15	It is not easy to skip a crucial step in proper use of the device.	1 2 3 4 5 N/A
16	The product can be easily used in the right hand.	1 2 3 4 5 N/A
17	The product can be easily used in the left hand.	1 2 3 4 5 N/A
18	The product can be easily used in either hand.	1 2 3 4 5 N/A
19	The use of the product does not require passing scalpel with the blade exposed.	1 2 3 4 5 N/A
20	The handle is similar in size and weight to standard scalpel.	1 2 3 4 5 N/A
21	The scalpel handle has grips for stable handling.	1 2 3 4 5 N/A

Of the above questions, which three are the most important to your safety when using this product?

Are there other questions which you feel should be asked regarding the safety features of this product?

1 Quart Sharps Container

Device Description:
Clear living hinged lid with a variety of openings in different sizes for disposal of blood needles, lancets, butterfly tubing, and small syringes.
Clearly labeled with a biohazard symbol for quick identification of sharps disposal.

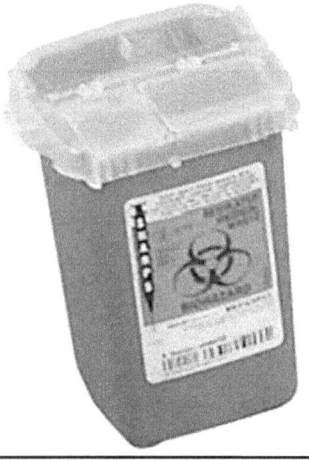

Advantages:
Unused containers nest inside each other to save storage space.
Compact enough to fit in trays and caddies.
Tamper resistant snap-on lids lock for final disposal.

Safety Features and Benefits:
Sealing gasket on lid guards against spills.

Mechanics:
1 quart - Available 100 per case or individually.

FDA Status:	N/A
Sizes Available:	1 quart -33/4"W x 6"H x 33/4"D
Product Website:	www.healthcarelogistics.com
Brochure Download:	www.healthcarelogistics.com
Instructional Website:	www.healthcarelogistics.com
Instructional Video:	www.healthcarelogistics.com
Availability:	Now available
Manufacturer:	Health Care Logistics 450 Town St Circleville, OH 43113 USA 740-477-1686 healthcarelogistics.com sottenweller@healthcarelogistics.com

Health Care Logistics INC. Your small friend, indeed

Sharps Disposal Containers

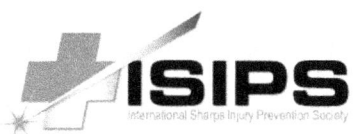

DISPOSABLE SHARPS CONTAINER EVALUATION FORM

Date: _____ Department: _____
Occupation: _____ Product: _____ Number of times used: _____

Please **circle** the most appropriate answer for each question.
Not applicable (N/A) may be used if the question does not apply to this particular product.

The Disposable Sharps Container:		Agree.........Disagree
1	Is puncture-resistant as certified to ASTM: F 2132-01.	1 2 3 4 5 N/A
2	Has documented compliance with Federal, State and local regulations.	1 2 3 4 5 N/A
3	Is leakproof on sides and bottom and during handling, storage and transport.	1 2 3 4 5 N/A
4	Is clearly labeled or color coded in accord with OSHA Bloodborne Pathogen (BBP) Standard.	1 2 3 4 5 N/A
5	Has a self-explanatory purpose & design, easily understood by busy users.	
6	Allows single-handed sharps deposit from all desired directions.	1 2 3 4 5 N/A
7	Can be placed at appropriate height allowing clear view of access by user.	1 2 3 4 5 N/A
8	Can be placed as close as feasible to where sharps are used.	1 2 3 4 5 N/A
9	Does not incorporate the use of needle unwinders which is prohibited by OSHA guidelines.	1 2 3 4 5 N/A
10	Is capable of taking and holding the size and volume of sharps used.	1 2 3 4 5 N/A
11	Permits safe, simple, entanglement-free disposal of sharps.	1 2 3 4 5 N/A
12	Is available in special designs for specific environments (Labs, OR, ER, etc).	1 2 3 4 5 N/A
13	Has an easily observable fill-status indicator, visible prior to sharps disposal.	1 2 3 4 5 N/A
14	Is stable when placed on horizontal surfaces in accord with product labelling.	1 2 3 4 5 N/A
15	Is designed to prevent hands or fingers from entering the container.	1 2 3 4 5 N/A
16	Defeats waste removal when open.	1 2 3 4 5 N/A
17	Has access designed to minimize sharps bounce-out.	1 2 3 4 5 N/A
18	Is designed so as to minimize risk of overfilling.	1 2 3 4 5 N/A
19	Has a closure mechanism that will not allow sharps injury during engagement.	1 2 3 4 5 N/A
20	Is resistant to manual opening when final closure mechanism is engaged.	1 2 3 4 5 N/A
21	Has optional locking bracketry.	1 2 3 4 5 N/A
22	Is easy to assemble, if required, and product is easily stored/stacked	1 2 3 4 5 N/A
23	Has rugged mounting brackets that are easy to service and decontaminate.	1 2 3 4 5 N/A
24	The design of the product is intuitive and does not require extensive user training.	1 2 3 4 5 N/A
25	Has a handle above the fill line that allows safe carrying of full container.	1 2 3 4 5 N/A
26	Is autoclavable, if necessary.	1 2 3 4 5 N/A
27	Has a design and final disposal that is environmentally sound.	1 2 3 4 5 N/A

Additional Evaluator concerns or comments:_____

_____

Your License: Each copy of each section of the safety device evaluation workbook is licensed to be used by a single facility. Similar to a software license, if you have multiple locations, you must purchase a copy of each section of the workbook that you choose to include in your Exposure Prevention Plan including each location or department in which it is to be used. At present, the workbook sells for about fifty cents for each device with evaluation form, so the burden of purchasing separate copies for each location where it is to be implemented is minimal.

The purpose of this workbook is to shave hundreds of man-hours off of the job of creating a sharps injury prevention plan and give you a real chance at compliance. It is expected to save you thousands of dollars in labor costs and help you to produce an otherwise prohibitively time consuming section of your ECP in record time. This workbook contains important data about nearly three hundred devices that have been designed specifically for the prevention of sharps injuries. Additionally, it contains a set of device evaluation charts designed to simplify the device evaluation process. Many more than these 300 devices are currently on the market. Most of their manufacturers are working with us. As soon as the manufacturers of these additional devices join us and submit their newer devices for publication, we will make updates available.

NOTE: Using this workbook will not produce a complete exposure control plan. It is designed so that you can comply with the most onerous sections of the BBP Standard. We do not guarantee you will survive an OSHA audit to your satisfaction, should one occur. These books are simply tools to help you prepare for such an eventuality and to help you to do it faster, cheaper, and in an organized and presentable fashion. These workbooks facilitate the safety device evaluation part of your plan.

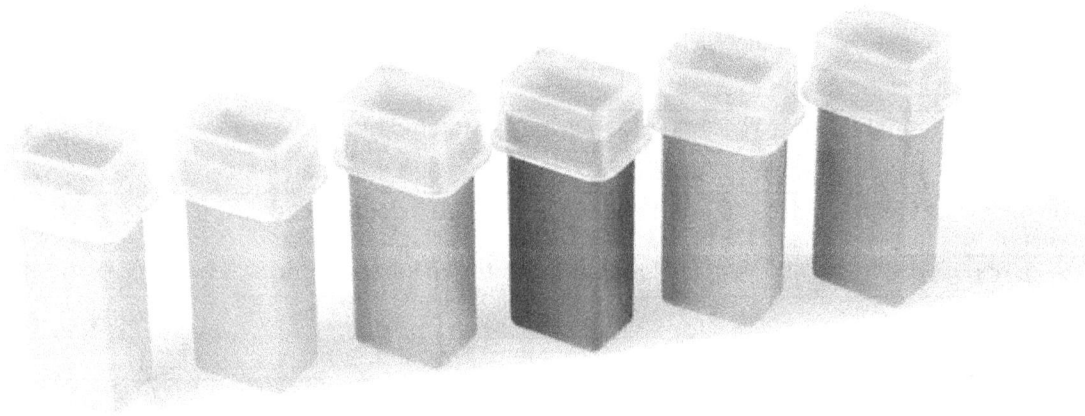

Again, our publication currently features nearly 300 devices, but there are still many more devices, probably around 400, that are on the market that are not yet included. These current editions include only the devices that have been listed with us by their manufacturers. The manufacturers have been notified and we plan to publish updates, with at least severty-five additional devices each, one or more times per year. We will keep you informed as additional devices are added to our database.

What is included with your purchase?

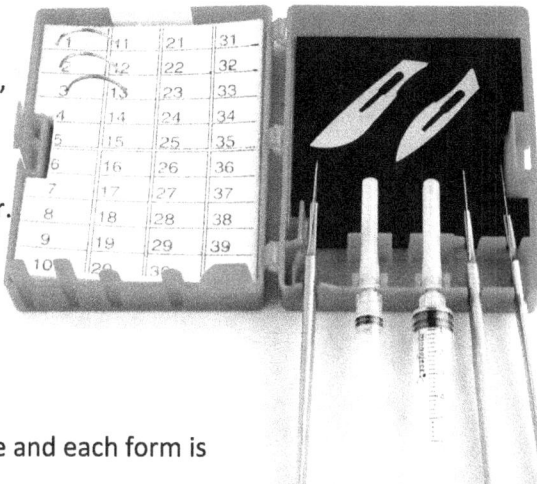

Book 1 includes a full set of evaluation forms before Section 1, and it includes your first installment of devices. Each of the devices has been paired with an evaluation form which was chosen by its manufacturer.

Book 2 includes sections 3 through 6.

Book 3 includes sections 7 through 9.

And **Book 4** includes sections 10 through 13.

Notice that each device is presented on a LEFT page and each form is presented on a right page, making it easy for most people to write on the page while seeing the device's presentation.

With your membership in MedicalSafetyDevices.com, you will always be just a click or two away from being able to order sample devices or additional literature. Never waste the time to make a phone call.

MedicalSafetyBook.com will do all that for you.

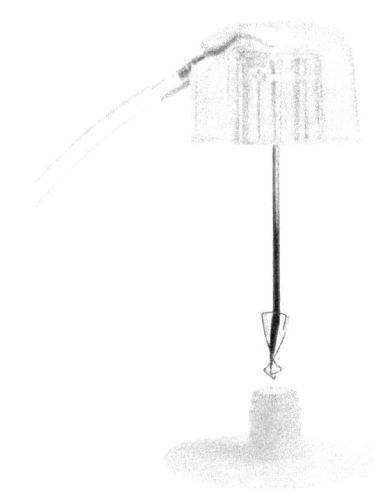

If you have an iPad, the sections are set up and organized to be saved as a category in iBooks.

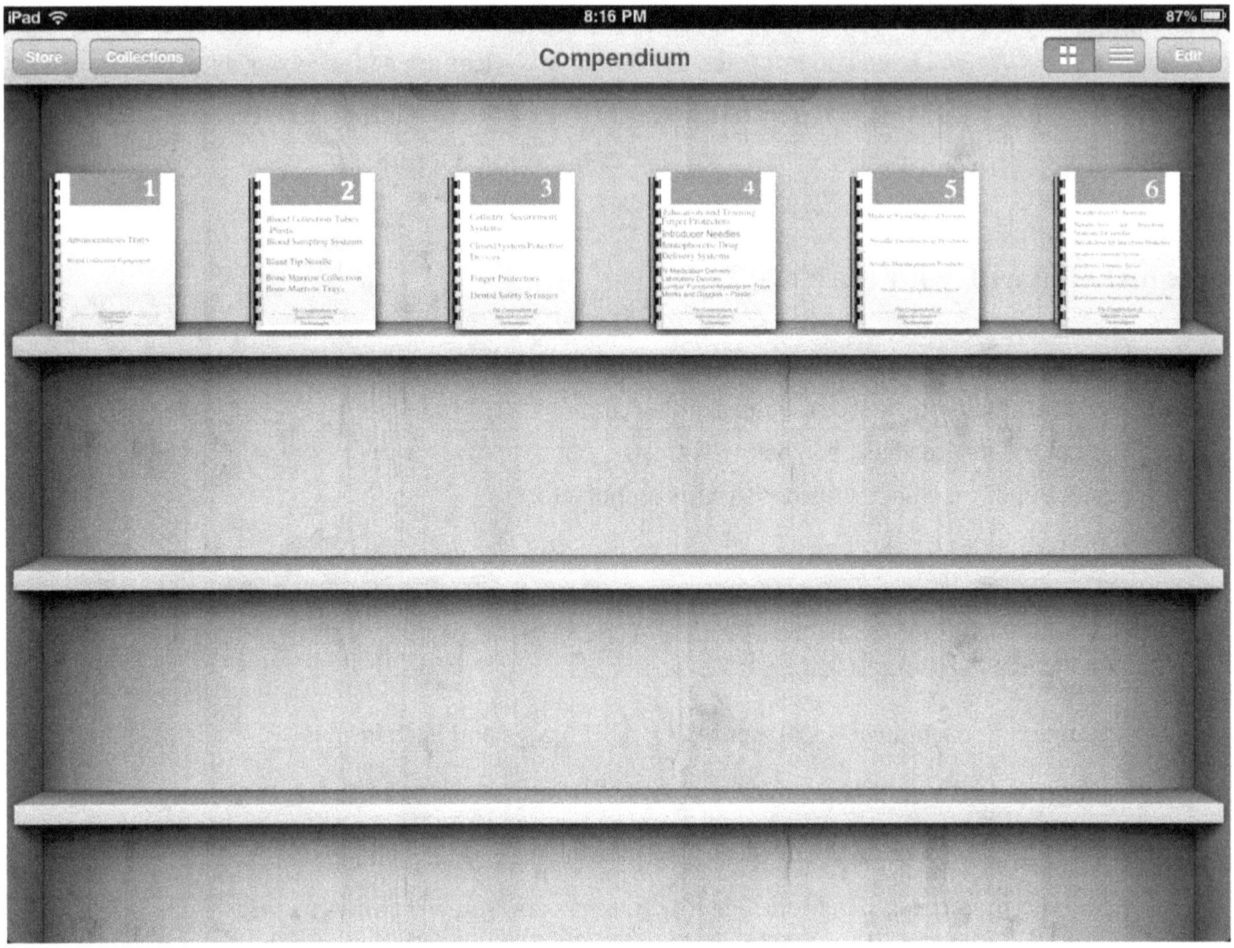

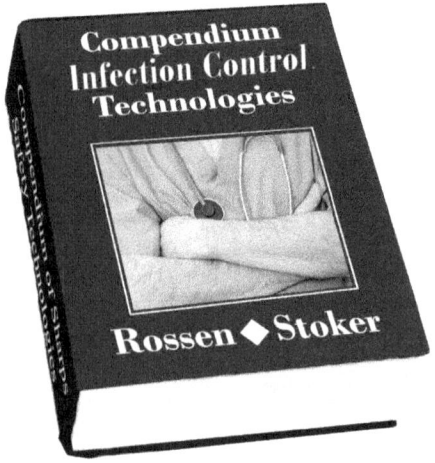

While now, only the printed versions are being released, as soon as the PDF versions of the workbook become available, they will be organized so as to be easily stored in the iBook format.

Above is a screen Capture of
iBooks bookshelf with the first six sections.

Categories of Devices

About 300 devices are included with the workbook. The following is a list of the various categories of devices that are covered in the 12 sections of this workbook. Although you will probably need all 12 sections, you can look over what is in each section and purchase what you decide you need.

Workbook - Book 1 includes sections 1 and 2

Section 1

<u>**Introduction**</u>

<u>**Forms for the Evaluation Of Safety Devices**</u>

<u>**Devices and Evaluation Forms**</u>

<u>**1. Amniocentesis Trays**</u>

<u>**2. Blood Collection Equipment**</u>

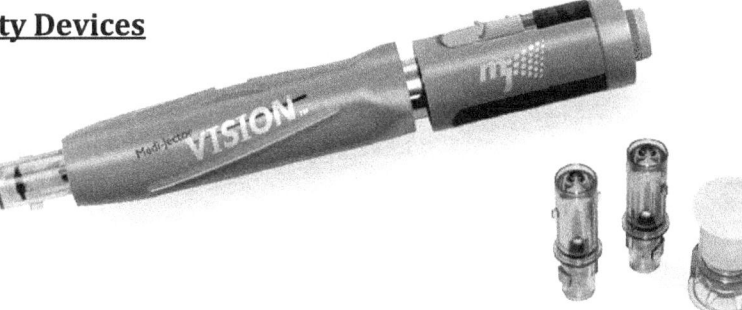

Section 2

<u>**3. Blood Collection Tubes - Plastic -**</u> <u>**4. Bone Marrow Collection**</u>

<u>**Systems**</u><u>**5. Bone Marrow Trays**</u>

<u>**6. Blunt Tip Needles**</u>

_____

Workbook - Book 2 includes sections 3-6

Section 3

<u>**7. Catheter Securement Systems**</u>

<u>**8. Closed System Protective Devices**</u>

<u>**9. Finger Protectors**</u>

<u>**10. Dental Safety Syringes**</u>

Section 4

Section 5

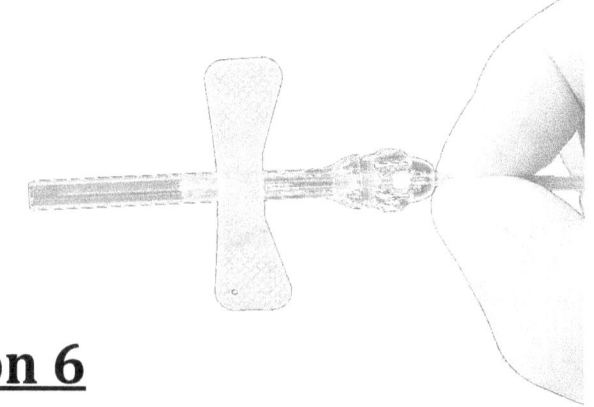

Section 6

Section 7

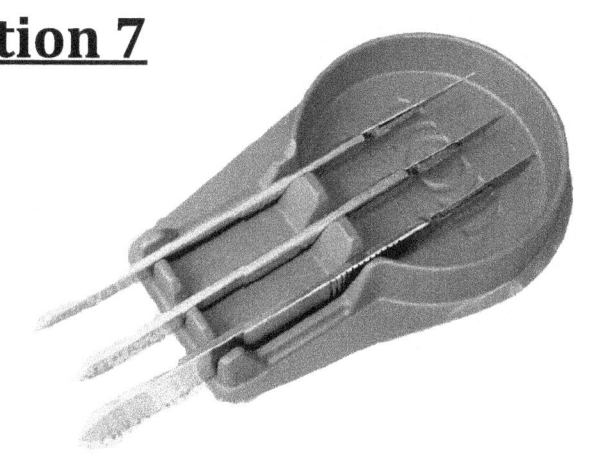

Section 8

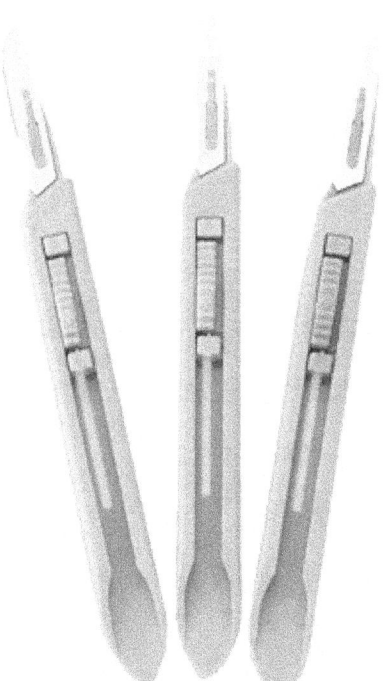

Section 9

_____

Section 10

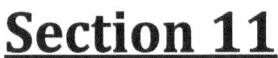

Section 11

Section 12

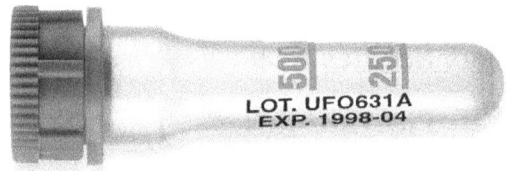

Continued next page

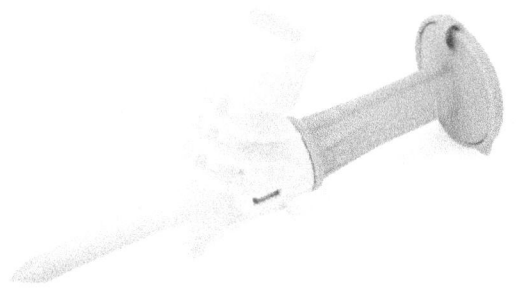

67. Vial Adapters

68. Wound Closure Technologies

69. Wound Irrigation

To continue building your ECP, go to Amazon.com and order Workbooks 1 through 4

NOTE: This is just the beginning. Books 5 - 8 are planned for the summer or fall of 2013. We have already identified an additional 400 devices that will be added as the year progresses.

At this time, we are simply waiting for those devices to be added to our database by their manufacturers. Most of the manufacturers are already members of MedicalSafetyBook.com and therefore we expect the progress of the next editions to be rather rapid.

We will release an update every time 100 or so additional devices are ready to print.

Make sure that you *go to MedicalSafetyBook.com and join.* Then we will not only let you know every time an update is ready, we will also email you each time a new device enters the database, so you will not necessarily have to wait for the next edition to continue working on your ECP.

Membership at MedicalSafetyBook.com is free. There you will have access to hundreds of free and low-priced samples and additional literature about the devices.

Just click on any device that you are considering or want samples of, and we will connect you and the manufacturers by email with just one click.

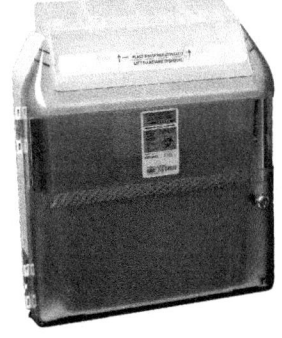
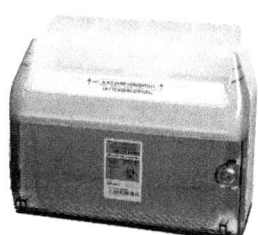